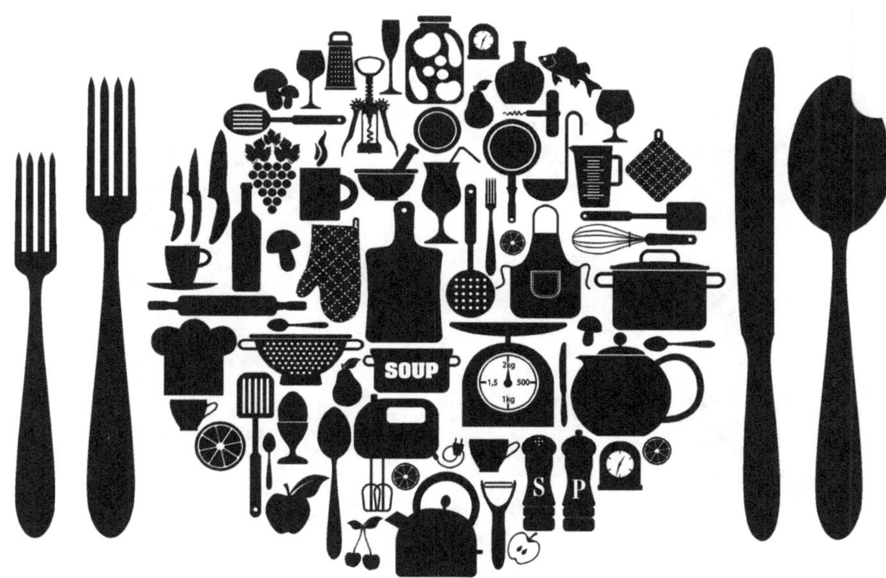

This Planner Belongs To:

Name : _______________________________

Nickname : _______________________________

Age : _______________________________

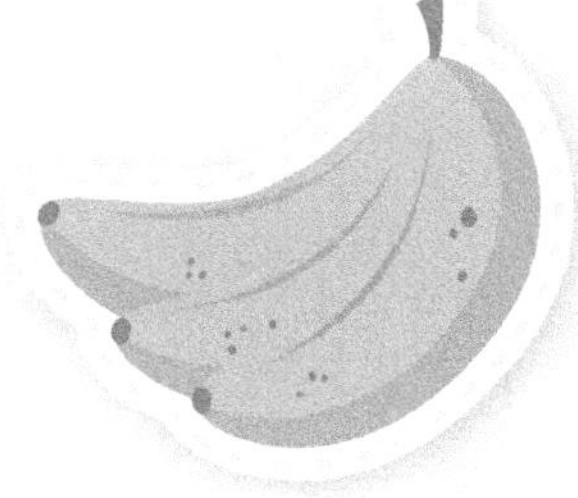

DAYS________________ DATE________________________ WEIGHT________________

Sleep (Hrs) : ☐ ☐ ☐ ☐ ☐ ☐ ☐ ☐ ☐ ☐
1 2 3 4 5 6 7 8 9 10 ....

Water (Cup) : ☐ ☐ ☐ ☐ ☐ ☐ ☐ ☐ ☐ ☐
1 2 3 4 5 6 7 8 9 10 ....

BREAKFAST	Calories	Carbs (g.)	Added Sugar (g.)	Fiber (g.)	Protein (g.)	Fat (g.)
Time _______ Total:						

SNACK						
Time _______ Total:						

LUNCH						
Time _______ Total:						

DINNER						
Time _______ Total:						

SNACK						
Time _______ Total:						

VITAMINS/SUPPLEMENT/MEDS	Notes

DAYS_____________________ **DATE**_______________________________ **WEIGHT**_______________

Sleep (Hrs) : ☐ ☐ ☐ ☐ ☐ ☐ ☐ ☐ ☐ ☐   Water (Cup) : ☐ ☐ ☐ ☐ ☐ ☐ ☐ ☐ ☐ ☐
         1   2   3   4   5   6   7   8   9   10   1   2   3   4   5   6   7   8   9   10 .....

BREAKFAST	Calories	Carbs (g.)	Added Sugar (g.)	Fiber (g.)	Protein (g.)	Fat (g.)
Time *Total:*						
SNACK						
Time *Total:*						
LUNCH						
Time *Total:*						
DINNER						
Time *Total:*						
SNACK						
Time *Total:*						

VITAMINS/SUPPLEMENT/MEDS	**Notes**

DAYS________________ **DATE**________________________ **WEIGHT**________________

Sleep (Hrs) : ☐ ☐ ☐ ☐ ☐ ☐ ☐ ☐ ☐ ☐ .....
           1 2 3 4 5 6 7 8 9 10

Water (Cup) : ☐ ☐ ☐ ☐ ☐ ☐ ☐ ☐ ☐ ☐ .....
            1 2 3 4 5 6 7 8 9 10

BREAKFAST	Calories	Carbs (g.)	Added Sugar (g.)	Fiber (g.)	Protein (g.)	Fat (g.)
Time _Total:_						

SNACK						
Time _Total:_						

LUNCH						
Time _Total:_						

DINNER						
Time _Total:_						

SNACK						
Time _Total:_						

VITAMINS/SUPPLEMENT/MEDS	Notes

DAYS__________________**DATE**___________________________ **WEIGHT**________________

Sleep (Hrs) : ☐ ☐ ☐ ☐ ☐ ☐ ☐ ☐ ☐ ☐
1 2 3 4 5 6 7 8 9 10 ....

Water (Cup) : ☐ ☐ ☐ ☐ ☐ ☐ ☐ ☐ ☐ ☐
1 2 3 4 5 6 7 8 9 10 ....

BREAKFAST	Calories	Carbs (g.)	Added Sugar (g.)	Fiber (g.)	Protein (g.)	Fat (g.)
Time	Total:					
SNACK						
Time	Total:					
LUNCH						
Time	Total:					
DINNER						
Time	Total:					
SNACK						
Time	Total:					

VITAMINS/SUPPLEMENT/MEDS	Notes

DAYS_________________**DATE**_____________________________**WEIGHT**_________________

Sleep (Hrs) : ☐ ☐ ☐ ☐ ☐ ☐ ☐ ☐ ☐ ☐
          1 2 3 4 5 6 7 8 9 10 .....

Water (Cup) : ☐ ☐ ☐ ☐ ☐ ☐ ☐ ☐ ☐ ☐
          1 2 3 4 5 6 7 8 9 10 .....

BREAKFAST	Calories	Carbs (g.)	Added Sugar (g.)	Fiber (g.)	Protein (g.)	Fat (g.)
Time *Total:*						

SNACK						
Time *Total:*						

LUNCH						
Time *Total:*						

DINNER						
Time *Total:*						

SNACK						
Time *Total:*						

VITAMINS/SUPPLEMENT/MEDS	Notes

DAYS______________ **DATE**______________________________ **WEIGHT**________________

Sleep (Hrs) : ☐ ☐ ☐ ☐ ☐ ☐ ☐ ☐ ☐ ☐   Water (Cup) : ☐ ☐ ☐ ☐ ☐ ☐ ☐ ☐ ☐ ☐
1 2 3 4 5 6 7 8 9 10 .....   1 2 3 4 5 6 7 8 9 10 .....

BREAKFAST	Calories	Carbs (g.)	Added Sugar (g.)	Fiber (g.)	Protein (g.)	Fat (g.)
Time Total:						
SNACK						
Time Total:						
LUNCH						
Time Total:						
DINNER						
Time Total:						
SNACK						
Time Total:						

VITAMINS/SUPPLEMENT/MEDS	Notes

DAYS_________________**DATE**_____________________________**WEIGHT**__________________

Sleep (Hrs) : ☐ ☐ ☐ ☐ ☐ ☐ ☐ ☐ ☐ ☐   Water (Cup) : ☐ ☐ ☐ ☐ ☐ ☐ ☐ ☐ ☐ ☐
         1 2 3 4 5 6 7 8 9 10 .....   1 2 3 4 5 6 7 8 9 10 .....

BREAKFAST	Calories	Carbs (g.)	Added Sugar (g.)	Fiber (g.)	Protein (g.)	Fat (g.)
Time _______ Total:						
SNACK						
Time _______ Total:						
LUNCH						
Time _______ Total:						
DINNER						
Time _______ Total:						
SNACK						
Time _______ Total:						

VITAMINS/SUPPLEMENT/MEDS	Notes

DAYS___________________**DATE**_____________________________**WEIGHT**_________________

Sleep (Hrs) : ☐ ☐ ☐ ☐ ☐ ☐ ☐ ☐ ☐ ☐
          1 2 3 4 5 6 7 8 9 10 .....

Water (Cup) : ☐ ☐ ☐ ☐ ☐ ☐ ☐ ☐ ☐ ☐
          1 2 3 4 5 6 7 8 9 10 .....

BREAKFAST	Calories	Carbs (g.)	Added Sugar (g.)	Fiber (g.)	Protein (g.)	Fat (g.)
Time *Total:*						
SNACK						
Time *Total:*						
LUNCH						
Time *Total:*						
DINNER						
Time *Total:*						
SNACK						
Time *Total:*						

VITAMINS/SUPPLEMENT/MEDS	Notes

DAYS_____________________**DATE**_______________________________**WEIGHT**_________________

Sleep (Hrs) : ☐ ☐ ☐ ☐ ☐ ☐ ☐ ☐ ☐ ☐   Water (Cup) : ☐ ☐ ☐ ☐ ☐ ☐ ☐ ☐ ☐ ☐
1 2 3 4 5 6 7 8 9 10 .....   1 2 3 4 5 6 7 8 9 10 .....

BREAKFAST	Calories	Carbs (g.)	Added Sugar (g.)	Fiber (g.)	Protein (g.)	Fat (g.)
Time *Total:*						

SNACK						
Time *Total:*						

LUNCH						
Time *Total:*						

DINNER						
Time *Total:*						

SNACK						
Time *Total:*						

VITAMINS/SUPPLEMENT/MEDS	Notes

DAYS______________________ **DATE**___________________________________ **WEIGHT**___________________

Sleep (Hrs) : ☐ ☐ ☐ ☐ ☐ ☐ ☐ ☐ ☐ ☐ .....
             1   2   3   4   5   6   7   8   9   10

Water (Cup) : ☐ ☐ ☐ ☐ ☐ ☐ ☐ ☐ ☐ ☐ .....
              1   2   3   4   5   6   7   8   9   10

BREAKFAST	Calories	Carbs (g.)	Added Sugar (g.)	Fiber (g.)	Protein (g.)	Fat (g.)
Time Total:						

SNACK	Calories	Carbs (g.)	Added Sugar (g.)	Fiber (g.)	Protein (g.)	Fat (g.)
Time Total:						

LUNCH	Calories	Carbs (g.)	Added Sugar (g.)	Fiber (g.)	Protein (g.)	Fat (g.)
Time Total:						

DINNER	Calories	Carbs (g.)	Added Sugar (g.)	Fiber (g.)	Protein (g.)	Fat (g.)
Time Total:						

SNACK	Calories	Carbs (g.)	Added Sugar (g.)	Fiber (g.)	Protein (g.)	Fat (g.)
Time Total:						

VITAMINS/SUPPLEMENT/MEDS	Notes

DAYS_________________ **DATE**_____________________________ **WEIGHT**___________________

Sleep (Hrs) : ☐ ☐ ☐ ☐ ☐ ☐ ☐ ☐ ☐ ☐   Water (Cup) : ☐ ☐ ☐ ☐ ☐ ☐ ☐ ☐ ☐ ☐
     1 2 3 4 5 6 7 8 9 10 .....   1 2 3 4 5 6 7 8 9 10 .....

BREAKFAST	Calories	Carbs (g.)	Added Sugar (g.)	Fiber (g.)	Protein (g.)	Fat (g.)
Time *Total:*						
SNACK						
Time *Total:*						
LUNCH						
Time *Total:*						
DINNER						
Time *Total:*						
SNACK						
Time *Total:*						

VITAMINS/SUPPLEMENT/MEDS	Notes

DAYS_________________**DATE**_____________________________**WEIGHT**_______________

Sleep (Hrs) : ☐ ☐ ☐ ☐ ☐ ☐ ☐ ☐ ☐ ☐
　　　　　　　1　2　3　4　5　6　7　8　9　10 .....

Water (Cup) : ☐ ☐ ☐ ☐ ☐ ☐ ☐ ☐ ☐ ☐
　　　　　　　1　2　3　4　5　6　7　8　9　10 .....

BREAKFAST	Calories	Carbs (g.)	Added Sugar (g.)	Fiber (g.)	Protein (g.)	Fat (g.)
Time — Total:						
SNACK						
Time — Total:						
LUNCH						
Time — Total:						
DINNER						
Time — Total:						
SNACK						
Time — Total:						

VITAMINS/SUPPLEMENT/MEDS	Notes

DAYS_________________**DATE**_______________________________**WEIGHT**_________________

Sleep (Hrs) : ☐ ☐ ☐ ☐ ☐ ☐ ☐ ☐ ☐ ☐   Water (Cup) : ☐ ☐ ☐ ☐ ☐ ☐ ☐ ☐ ☐ ☐
           1   2   3   4   5   6   7   8   9   10   1   2   3   4   5   6   7   8   9   10 .....

BREAKFAST	Calories	Carbs (g.)	Added Sugar (g.)	Fiber (g.)	Protein (g.)	Fat (g.)
Time *Total:*						
SNACK						
Time *Total:*						
LUNCH						
Time *Total:*						
DINNER						
Time *Total:*						
SNACK						
Time *Total:*						

VITAMINS/SUPPLEMENT/MEDS	Notes

DAYS______________________**DATE**______________________________ **WEIGHT**________________

Sleep (Hrs) : ☐ ☐ ☐ ☐ ☐ ☐ ☐ ☐ ☐ ☐   Water (Cup) : ☐ ☐ ☐ ☐ ☐ ☐ ☐ ☐ ☐ ☐
           1 2 3 4 5 6 7 8 9 10 .....   1 2 3 4 5 6 7 8 9 10 .....

BREAKFAST	Calories	Carbs (g.)	Added Sugar (g.)	Fiber (g.)	Protein (g.)	Fat (g.)
Time *Total:*						
SNACK						
Time *Total:*						
LUNCH						
Time *Total:*						
DINNER						
Time *Total:*						
SNACK						
Time *Total:*						

VITAMINS/SUPPLEMENT/MEDS	**Notes**

DAYS______________________**DATE**__________________________________**WEIGHT**__________________

Sleep (Hrs) : ☐ ☐ ☐ ☐ ☐ ☐ ☐ ☐ ☐ ☐ ......   Water (Cup) : ☐ ☐ ☐ ☐ ☐ ☐ ☐ ☐ ☐ ☐ ......
          1   2   3   4   5   6   7   8   9   10   1   2   3   4   5   6   7   8   9   10

BREAKFAST	Calories	Carbs (g.)	Added Sugar (g.)	Fiber (g.)	Protein (g.)	Fat (g.)
Time *Total:*						
SNACK						
Time *Total:*						
LUNCH						
Time *Total:*						
DINNER						
Time *Total:*						
SNACK						
Time *Total:*						

VITAMINS/SUPPLEMENT/MEDS	Notes

DAYS______________________ **DATE**______________________________ **WEIGHT**________________________

Sleep (Hrs) : ☐ ☐ ☐ ☐ ☐ ☐ ☐ ☐ ☐ ☐
1 2 3 4 5 6 7 8 9 10 .....

Water (Cup) : ☐ ☐ ☐ ☐ ☐ ☐ ☐ ☐ ☐ ☐
1 2 3 4 5 6 7 8 9 10 .....

BREAKFAST	Calories	Carbs (g.)	Added Sugar (g.)	Fiber (g.)	Protein (g.)	Fat (g.)
Time Total:						

SNACK						
Time Total:						

LUNCH						
Time Total:						

DINNER						
Time Total:						

SNACK						
Time Total:						

VITAMINS/SUPPLEMENT/MEDS	Notes

DAYS_____________________ **DATE**_____________________________ **WEIGHT**_________________

Sleep (Hrs) : ☐ ☐ ☐ ☐ ☐ ☐ ☐ ☐ ☐ ☐   Water (Cup) : ☐ ☐ ☐ ☐ ☐ ☐ ☐ ☐ ☐ ☐
             1 2 3 4 5 6 7 8 9 10 .....   1 2 3 4 5 6 7 8 9 10 .....

BREAKFAST	Calories	Carbs (g.)	Added Sugar (g.)	Fiber (g.)	Protein (g.)	Fat (g.)
Time *Total:*						
SNACK						
Time *Total:*						
LUNCH						
Time *Total:*						
DINNER						
Time *Total:*						
SNACK						
Time *Total:*						

VITAMINS/SUPPLEMENT/MEDS	**Notes**

DAYS__________________**DATE**______________________________**WEIGHT**__________________

Sleep (Hrs) : ☐ ☐ ☐ ☐ ☐ ☐ ☐ ☐ ☐ ☐   Water (Cup) : ☐ ☐ ☐ ☐ ☐ ☐ ☐ ☐ ☐ ☐
1   2   3   4   5   6   7   8   9   10   1   2   3   4   5   6   7   8   9   10 .....

BREAKFAST	Calories	Carbs (g.)	Added Sugar (g.)	Fiber (g.)	Protein (g.)	Fat (g.)
Time *Total:*						
SNACK						
Time *Total:*						
LUNCH						
Time *Total:*						
DINNER						
Time *Total:*						
SNACK						
Time *Total:*						

VITAMINS/SUPPLEMENT/MEDS	Notes

DAYS______________________**DATE**________________________________**WEIGHT**________________________

Sleep (Hrs) : ☐ ☐ ☐ ☐ ☐ ☐ ☐ ☐ ☐ ☐   Water (Cup) : ☐ ☐ ☐ ☐ ☐ ☐ ☐ ☐ ☐ ☐
        1 2 3 4 5 6 7 8 9 10 .....   1 2 3 4 5 6 7 8 9 10 .....

BREAKFAST	Calories	Carbs (g.)	Added Sugar (g.)	Fiber (g.)	Protein (g.)	Fat (g.)
Time *Total:*						

SNACK						
Time *Total:*						

LUNCH						
Time *Total:*						

DINNER						
Time *Total:*						

SNACK						
Time *Total:*						

VITAMINS/SUPPLEMENT/MEDS	Notes

DAYS_________________ **DATE**_________________________________ **WEIGHT**_______________

Sleep (Hrs) : ☐ ☐ ☐ ☐ ☐ ☐ ☐ ☐ ☐ ☐
1　2　3　4　5　6　7　8　9　10 .....

Water (Cup) : ☐ ☐ ☐ ☐ ☐ ☐ ☐ ☐ ☐ ☐
1　2　3　4　5　6　7　8　9　10 .....

BREAKFAST	Calories	Carbs (g.)	Added Sugar (g.)	Fiber (g.)	Protein (g.)	Fat (g.)
Time _______ Total:						

SNACK						
Time _______ Total:						

LUNCH						
Time _______ Total:						

DINNER						
Time _______ Total:						

SNACK						
Time _______ Total:						

VITAMINS/SUPPLEMENT/MEDS	Notes

DAYS______________________**DATE**______________________________________**WEIGHT**__________________

Sleep (Hrs) : ☐ ☐ ☐ ☐ ☐ ☐ ☐ ☐ ☐ ☐
          1 2 3 4 5 6 7 8 9 10 .....

Water (Cup) : ☐ ☐ ☐ ☐ ☐ ☐ ☐ ☐ ☐ ☐
           1 2 3 4 5 6 7 8 9 10 .....

BREAKFAST	Calories	Carbs (g.)	Added Sugar (g.)	Fiber (g.)	Protein (g.)	Fat (g.)
Time *Total:*						
SNACK						
Time *Total:*						
LUNCH						
Time *Total:*						
DINNER						
Time *Total:*						
SNACK						
Time *Total:*						

VITAMINS/SUPPLEMENT/MEDS	Notes

DAYS_______________ **DATE**_________________________________ **WEIGHT**_______________

Sleep (Hrs) : ☐ ☐ ☐ ☐ ☐ ☐ ☐ ☐ ☐ ☐   Water (Cup) : ☐ ☐ ☐ ☐ ☐ ☐ ☐ ☐ ☐ ☐
        1   2   3   4   5   6   7   8   9   10   1   2   3   4   5   6   7   8   9   10 .....

BREAKFAST	Calories	Carbs (g.)	Added Sugar (g.)	Fiber (g.)	Protein (g.)	Fat (g.)
Time	Total:					
SNACK						
Time	Total:					
LUNCH						
Time	Total:					
DINNER						
Time	Total:					
SNACK						
Time	Total:					

VITAMINS/SUPPLEMENT/MEDS	Notes

DAYS______________**DATE**________________________**WEIGHT**________________

Sleep (Hrs) : ☐ ☐ ☐ ☐ ☐ ☐ ☐ ☐ ☐ ☐
          1   2   3   4   5   6   7   8   9   10 .....

Water (Cup) : ☐ ☐ ☐ ☐ ☐ ☐ ☐ ☐ ☐ ☐
          1   2   3   4   5   6   7   8   9   10 .....

BREAKFAST	Calories	Carbs (g.)	Added Sugar (g.)	Fiber (g.)	Protein (g.)	Fat (g.)
Time *Total:*						
SNACK						
Time *Total:*						
LUNCH						
Time *Total:*						
DINNER						
Time *Total:*						
SNACK						
Time *Total:*						

VITAMINS/SUPPLEMENT/MEDS	Notes

DAYS______________ **DATE**______________________ **WEIGHT**______________

Sleep (Hrs) : ☐ ☐ ☐ ☐ ☐ ☐ ☐ ☐ ☐ ☐   Water (Cup) : ☐ ☐ ☐ ☐ ☐ ☐ ☐ ☐ ☐ ☐
            1   2   3   4   5   6   7   8   9   10   1   2   3   4   5   6   7   8   9   10 .....

BREAKFAST	Calories	Carbs (g.)	Added Sugar (g.)	Fiber (g.)	Protein (g.)	Fat (g.)
Time *Total:*						
SNACK						
Time *Total:*						
LUNCH						
Time *Total:*						
DINNER						
Time *Total:*						
SNACK						
Time *Total:*						

VITAMINS/SUPPLEMENT/MEDS	Notes

DAYS__________________**DATE**______________________________**WEIGHT**__________________

Sleep (Hrs) : ☐ ☐ ☐ ☐ ☐ ☐ ☐ ☐ ☐ ☐   Water (Cup) : ☐ ☐ ☐ ☐ ☐ ☐ ☐ ☐ ☐ ☐
       1 2 3 4 5 6 7 8 9 10 .....   1 2 3 4 5 6 7 8 9 10 .....

BREAKFAST	Calories	Carbs (g.)	Added Sugar (g.)	Fiber (g.)	Protein (g.)	Fat (g.)
Time *Total:*						
SNACK						
Time *Total:*						
LUNCH						
Time *Total:*						
DINNER						
Time *Total:*						
SNACK						
Time *Total:*						

VITAMINS/SUPPLEMENT/MEDS	Notes

DAYS_________________ **DATE**_________________________________ **WEIGHT**___________________

Sleep (Hrs) : ☐ ☐ ☐ ☐ ☐ ☐ ☐ ☐ ☐ ☐
         1 2 3 4 5 6 7 8 9 10 .....

Water (Cup) : ☐ ☐ ☐ ☐ ☐ ☐ ☐ ☐ ☐ ☐
         1 2 3 4 5 6 7 8 9 10 .....

BREAKFAST	Calories	Carbs (g.)	Added Sugar (g.)	Fiber (g.)	Protein (g.)	Fat (g.)
Time *Total:*						
SNACK						
Time *Total:*						
LUNCH						
Time *Total:*						
DINNER						
Time *Total:*						
SNACK						
Time *Total:*						

VITAMINS/SUPPLEMENT/MEDS	Notes

DAYS___________________ **DATE**_____________________________ **WEIGHT**_________________

Sleep (Hrs) : ☐ ☐ ☐ ☐ ☐ ☐ ☐ ☐ ☐ ☐   Water (Cup) : ☐ ☐ ☐ ☐ ☐ ☐ ☐ ☐ ☐ ☐
1 2 3 4 5 6 7 8 9 10 .....   1 2 3 4 5 6 7 8 9 10 .....

BREAKFAST	Calories	Carbs (g.)	Added Sugar (g.)	Fiber (g.)	Protein (g.)	Fat (g.)
Time *Total:*						
SNACK						
Time *Total:*						
LUNCH						
Time *Total:*						
DINNER						
Time *Total:*						
SNACK						
Time *Total:*						

VITAMINS/SUPPLEMENT/MEDS	Notes

DAYS___________________ **DATE**_________________________________ **WEIGHT**__________________

Sleep (Hrs) : ☐ ☐ ☐ ☐ ☐ ☐ ☐ ☐ ☐ ☐
1 2 3 4 5 6 7 8 9 10 ....

Water (Cup) : ☐ ☐ ☐ ☐ ☐ ☐ ☐ ☐ ☐ ☐
1 2 3 4 5 6 7 8 9 10 ....

BREAKFAST	Calories	Carbs (g.)	Added Sugar (g.)	Fiber (g.)	Protein (g.)	Fat (g.)
Time Total:						
SNACK						
Time Total:						
LUNCH						
Time Total:						
DINNER						
Time Total:						
SNACK						
Time Total:						

VITAMINS/SUPPLEMENT/MEDS	Notes

DAYS________________________**DATE**_________________________________**WEIGHT**________________________

Sleep (Hrs) : ☐ ☐ ☐ ☐ ☐ ☐ ☐ ☐ ☐ ☐   Water (Cup) : ☐ ☐ ☐ ☐ ☐ ☐ ☐ ☐ ☐ ☐
      1 2 3 4 5 6 7 8 9 10 .....   1 2 3 4 5 6 7 8 9 10 .....

BREAKFAST	Calories	Carbs (g.)	Added Sugar (g.)	Fiber (g.)	Protein (g.)	Fat (g.)
Time *Total:*						
SNACK						
Time *Total:*						
LUNCH						
Time *Total:*						
DINNER						
Time *Total:*						
SNACK						
Time *Total:*						

VITAMINS/SUPPLEMENT/MEDS	Notes

DAYS___________________ **DATE**_______________________________ **WEIGHT**___________________

Sleep (Hrs) : ☐ ☐ ☐ ☐ ☐ ☐ ☐ ☐ ☐ ☐ .....   Water (Cup) : ☐ ☐ ☐ ☐ ☐ ☐ ☐ ☐ ☐ ☐ .....
             1 2 3 4 5 6 7 8 9 10

BREAKFAST	Calories	Carbs (g.)	Added Sugar (g.)	Fiber (g.)	Protein (g.)	Fat (g.)
Time Total:						
SNACK						
Time Total:						
LUNCH						
Time Total:						
DINNER						
Time Total:						
SNACK						
Time Total:						

VITAMINS/SUPPLEMENT/MEDS	Notes

DAYS_______________________**DATE**______________________________**WEIGHT**________________

Sleep (Hrs) : ☐ ☐ ☐ ☐ ☐ ☐ ☐ ☐ ☐ ☐   Water (Cup) : ☐ ☐ ☐ ☐ ☐ ☐ ☐ ☐ ☐ ☐
      1 2 3 4 5 6 7 8 9 10 .....   1 2 3 4 5 6 7 8 9 10 .....

BREAKFAST	Calories	Carbs (g.)	Added Sugar (g.)	Fiber (g.)	Protein (g.)	Fat (g.)
Time *Total:*						
SNACK						
Time *Total:*						
LUNCH						
Time *Total:*						
DINNER						
Time *Total:*						
SNACK						
Time *Total:*						

VITAMINS/SUPPLEMENT/MEDS	Notes

DAYS________________ **DATE**________________________ **WEIGHT**________________

Sleep (Hrs) : ☐ ☐ ☐ ☐ ☐ ☐ ☐ ☐ ☐ ☐   Water (Cup) : ☐ ☐ ☐ ☐ ☐ ☐ ☐ ☐ ☐ ☐
  1 2 3 4 5 6 7 8 9 10 .....   1 2 3 4 5 6 7 8 9 10 .....

BREAKFAST	Calories	Carbs (g.)	Added Sugar (g.)	Fiber (g.)	Protein (g.)	Fat (g.)
Time Total:						
SNACK						
Time Total:						
LUNCH						
Time Total:						
DINNER						
Time Total:						
SNACK						
Time Total:						

VITAMINS/SUPPLEMENT/MEDS	Notes

DAYS___________________**DATE**___________________________________**WEIGHT**_________________

Sleep (Hrs) : ☐ ☐ ☐ ☐ ☐ ☐ ☐ ☐ ☐ ☐ .....   Water (Cup) : ☐ ☐ ☐ ☐ ☐ ☐ ☐ ☐ ☐ ☐ .....
1 2 3 4 5 6 7 8 9 10   1 2 3 4 5 6 7 8 9 10

BREAKFAST	Calories	Carbs (g.)	Added Sugar (g.)	Fiber (g.)	Protein (g.)	Fat (g.)
Time *Total:*						
SNACK						
Time *Total:*						
LUNCH						
Time *Total:*						
DINNER						
Time *Total:*						
SNACK						
Time *Total:*						

VITAMINS/SUPPLEMENT/MEDS	Notes

DAYS______________ **DATE**________________________________ **WEIGHT**______________

Sleep (Hrs) : ☐ ☐ ☐ ☐ ☐ ☐ ☐ ☐ ☐ ☐ Water (Cup) : ☐ ☐ ☐ ☐ ☐ ☐ ☐ ☐ ☐ ☐
          1   2   3   4   5   6   7   8   9   10   1   2   3   4   5   6   7   8   9   10 .....

BREAKFAST	Calories	Carbs (g.)	Added Sugar (g.)	Fiber (g.)	Protein (g.)	Fat (g.)
Time	Total:					
SNACK						
Time	Total:					
LUNCH						
Time	Total:					
DINNER						
Time	Total:					
SNACK						
Time	Total:					

VITAMINS/SUPPLEMENT/MEDS	Notes

DAYS_______________ **DATE**_______________________ **WEIGHT**_______________

Sleep (Hrs) : ☐ ☐ ☐ ☐ ☐ ☐ ☐ ☐ ☐ ☐
          1 2 3 4 5 6 7 8 9 10 .....

Water (Cup) : ☐ ☐ ☐ ☐ ☐ ☐ ☐ ☐ ☐ ☐
           1 2 3 4 5 6 7 8 9 10 .....

BREAKFAST	Calories	Carbs (g.)	Added Sugar (g.)	Fiber (g.)	Protein (g.)	Fat (g.)
Time *Total:*						
SNACK						
Time *Total:*						
LUNCH						
Time *Total:*						
DINNER						
Time *Total:*						
SNACK						
Time *Total:*						

VITAMINS/SUPPLEMENT/MEDS	Notes

DAYS_____________________ **DATE**_________________________________ **WEIGHT**_____________________

Sleep (Hrs) : ☐ ☐ ☐ ☐ ☐ ☐ ☐ ☐ ☐ ☐ ....
         1 2 3 4 5 6 7 8 9 10

Water (Cup) : ☐ ☐ ☐ ☐ ☐ ☐ ☐ ☐ ☐ ☐ ....
         1 2 3 4 5 6 7 8 9 10

BREAKFAST	Calories	Carbs (g.)	Added Sugar (g.)	Fiber (g.)	Protein (g.)	Fat (g.)
Time *Total:*						
SNACK						
Time *Total:*						
LUNCH						
Time *Total:*						
DINNER						
Time *Total:*						
SNACK						
Time *Total:*						

VITAMINS/SUPPLEMENT/MEDS	**Notes**

DAYS________________**DATE**________________________**WEIGHT**________________

Sleep (Hrs) : ☐ ☐ ☐ ☐ ☐ ☐ ☐ ☐ ☐ ☐
               1 2 3 4 5 6 7 8 9 10 .....

Water (Cup) : ☐ ☐ ☐ ☐ ☐ ☐ ☐ ☐ ☐ ☐
                1 2 3 4 5 6 7 8 9 10 .....

BREAKFAST	Calories	Carbs (g.)	Added Sugar (g.)	Fiber (g.)	Protein (g.)	Fat (g.)
Time *Total:*						

SNACK						
Time *Total:*						

LUNCH						
Time *Total:*						

DINNER						
Time *Total:*						

SNACK						
Time *Total:*						

VITAMINS/SUPPLEMENT/MEDS	Notes

DAYS____________________ **DATE**________________________________ **WEIGHT**____________________

Sleep (Hrs) : ☐ ☐ ☐ ☐ ☐ ☐ ☐ ☐ ☐ ☐
          1 2 3 4 5 6 7 8 9 10 ....

Water (Cup) : ☐ ☐ ☐ ☐ ☐ ☐ ☐ ☐ ☐ ☐
          1 2 3 4 5 6 7 8 9 10 ....

BREAKFAST	Calories	Carbs (g.)	Added Sugar (g.)	Fiber (g.)	Protein (g.)	Fat (g.)
Time *Total:*						
SNACK						
Time *Total:*						
LUNCH						
Time *Total:*						
DINNER						
Time *Total:*						
SNACK						
Time *Total:*						

VITAMINS/SUPPLEMENT/MEDS	Notes

DAYS_______________**DATE**_____________________________**WEIGHT**_______________

Sleep (Hrs) : ☐ ☐ ☐ ☐ ☐ ☐ ☐ ☐ ☐ ☐
         1 2 3 4 5 6 7 8 9 10 .....

Water (Cup) : ☐ ☐ ☐ ☐ ☐ ☐ ☐ ☐ ☐ ☐
           1 2 3 4 5 6 7 8 9 10 .....

BREAKFAST	Calories	Carbs (g.)	Added Sugar (g.)	Fiber (g.)	Protein (g.)	Fat (g.)
Time *Total:*						
SNACK						
Time *Total:*						
LUNCH						
Time *Total:*						
DINNER						
Time *Total:*						
SNACK						
Time *Total:*						

VITAMINS/SUPPLEMENT/MEDS	Notes

DAYS_________________ **DATE**_________________________ **WEIGHT**_______________

Sleep (Hrs) : ☐ ☐ ☐ ☐ ☐ ☐ ☐ ☐ ☐ ☐
          1 2 3 4 5 6 7 8 9 10 ....

Water (Cup) : ☐ ☐ ☐ ☐ ☐ ☐ ☐ ☐ ☐ ☐
          1 2 3 4 5 6 7 8 9 10 ....

BREAKFAST	Calories	Carbs (g.)	Added Sugar (g.)	Fiber (g.)	Protein (g.)	Fat (g.)
Time Total:						
SNACK						
Time Total:						
LUNCH						
Time Total:						
DINNER						
Time Total:						
SNACK						
Time Total:						

VITAMINS/SUPPLEMENT/MEDS	Notes

DAYS____________________**DATE**____________________________________**WEIGHT**__________________

Sleep (Hrs) : ☐ ☐ ☐ ☐ ☐ ☐ ☐ ☐ ☐ ☐
          1 2 3 4 5 6 7 8 9 10 .....

Water (Cup) : ☐ ☐ ☐ ☐ ☐ ☐ ☐ ☐ ☐ ☐
          1 2 3 4 5 6 7 8 9 10 .....

BREAKFAST	Calories	Carbs (g.)	Added Sugar (g.)	Fiber (g.)	Protein (g.)	Fat (g.)
Time *Total:*						
SNACK						
Time *Total:*						
LUNCH						
Time *Total:*						
DINNER						
Time *Total:*						
SNACK						
Time *Total:*						

VITAMINS/SUPPLEMENT/MEDS	Notes

DAYS_________________ **DATE**_________________________________ **WEIGHT**_________________

Sleep (Hrs) : ☐ ☐ ☐ ☐ ☐ ☐ ☐ ☐ ☐ ☐
1 2 3 4 5 6 7 8 9 10 .....

Water (Cup) : ☐ ☐ ☐ ☐ ☐ ☐ ☐ ☐ ☐ ☐
1 2 3 4 5 6 7 8 9 10 .....

BREAKFAST	Calories	Carbs (g.)	Added Sugar (g.)	Fiber (g.)	Protein (g.)	Fat (g.)
Time *Total:*						

SNACK						
Time *Total:*						

LUNCH						
Time *Total:*						

DINNER						
Time *Total:*						

SNACK						
Time *Total:*						

VITAMINS/SUPPLEMENT/MEDS	Notes

DAYS_________________**DATE**_______________________________**WEIGHT**________________

Sleep (Hrs) : ☐ ☐ ☐ ☐ ☐ ☐ ☐ ☐ ☐ ☐ Water (Cup) : ☐ ☐ ☐ ☐ ☐ ☐ ☐ ☐ ☐ ☐
       1 2 3 4 5 6 7 8 9 10 .....   1 2 3 4 5 6 7 8 9 10 .....

BREAKFAST	Calories	Carbs (g.)	Added Sugar (g.)	Fiber (g.)	Protein (g.)	Fat (g.)
Time *Total:*						
SNACK						
Time *Total:*						
LUNCH						
Time *Total:*						
DINNER						
Time *Total:*						
SNACK						
Time *Total:*						

VITAMINS/SUPPLEMENT/MEDS	Notes

DAYS_______________**DATE**_______________________________**WEIGHT**_______________

Sleep (Hrs) : ☐ ☐ ☐ ☐ ☐ ☐ ☐ ☐ ☐ ☐
         1 2 3 4 5 6 7 8 9 10 ....

Water (Cup) : ☐ ☐ ☐ ☐ ☐ ☐ ☐ ☐ ☐ ☐
         1 2 3 4 5 6 7 8 9 10 ....

BREAKFAST	Calories	Carbs (g.)	Added Sugar (g.)	Fiber (g.)	Protein (g.)	Fat (g.)
Time Total:						
SNACK						
Time Total:						
LUNCH						
Time Total:						
DINNER						
Time Total:						
SNACK						
Time Total:						

VITAMINS/SUPPLEMENT/MEDS	Notes

DAYS___________________**DATE**___________________________**WEIGHT**_______________

Sleep (Hrs) : ☐ ☐ ☐ ☐ ☐ ☐ ☐ ☐ ☐ ☐
       1 2 3 4 5 6 7 8 9 10 .....

Water (Cup) : ☐ ☐ ☐ ☐ ☐ ☐ ☐ ☐ ☐ ☐
       1 2 3 4 5 6 7 8 9 10 .....

BREAKFAST	Calories	Carbs (g.)	Added Sugar (g.)	Fiber (g.)	Protein (g.)	Fat (g.)
Time *Total:*						

SNACK						
Time *Total:*						

LUNCH						
Time *Total:*						

DINNER						
Time *Total:*						

SNACK						
Time *Total:*						

VITAMINS/SUPPLEMENT/MEDS	Notes

DAYS_________________ **DATE**_________________________________ **WEIGHT**_________________

Sleep (Hrs) : ☐ ☐ ☐ ☐ ☐ ☐ ☐ ☐ ☐ ☐ ..... Water (Cup) : ☐ ☐ ☐ ☐ ☐ ☐ ☐ ☐ ☐ ☐ .....
         1 2 3 4 5 6 7 8 9 10   1 2 3 4 5 6 7 8 9 10

BREAKFAST	Calories	Carbs (g.)	Added Sugar (g.)	Fiber (g.)	Protein (g.)	Fat (g.)
Time _______ Total:						
SNACK						
Time _______ Total:						
LUNCH						
Time _______ Total:						
DINNER						
Time _______ Total:						
SNACK						
Time _______ Total:						

VITAMINS/SUPPLEMENT/MEDS	Notes

DAYS_____________________**DATE**_____________________________________**WEIGHT**_____________________

Sleep (Hrs) : ☐ ☐ ☐ ☐ ☐ ☐ ☐ ☐ ☐ ☐ .....
          1 2 3 4 5 6 7 8 9 10

Water (Cup) : ☐ ☐ ☐ ☐ ☐ ☐ ☐ ☐ ☐ ☐ .....
          1 2 3 4 5 6 7 8 9 10

BREAKFAST	Calories	Carbs (g.)	Added Sugar (g.)	Fiber (g.)	Protein (g.)	Fat (g.)
Time *Total:*						

SNACK						
Time *Total:*						

LUNCH						
Time *Total:*						

DINNER						
Time *Total:*						

SNACK						
Time *Total:*						

VITAMINS/SUPPLEMENT/MEDS	Notes

DAYS______________________**DATE**_______________________________**WEIGHT**________________

Sleep (Hrs) : ☐ ☐ ☐ ☐ ☐ ☐ ☐ ☐ ☐ ☐ .....
　　　　　　　1　2　3　4　5　6　7　8　9　10

Water (Cup) : ☐ ☐ ☐ ☐ ☐ ☐ ☐ ☐ ☐ ☐ .....
　　　　　　　　1　2　3　4　5　6　7　8　9　10

BREAKFAST	Calories	Carbs (g.)	Added Sugar (g.)	Fiber (g.)	Protein (g.)	Fat (g.)
Time　　　　　　　*Total:*						
SNACK						
Time　　　　　　　*Total:*						
LUNCH						
Time　　　　　　　*Total:*						
DINNER						
Time　　　　　　　*Total:*						
SNACK						
Time　　　　　　　*Total:*						

VITAMINS/SUPPLEMENT/MEDS	Notes

DAYS________________**DATE**________________________**WEIGHT**________________

Sleep (Hrs) : ☐ ☐ ☐ ☐ ☐ ☐ ☐ ☐ ☐ ☐
            1 2 3 4 5 6 7 8 9 10 .....

Water (Cup) : ☐ ☐ ☐ ☐ ☐ ☐ ☐ ☐ ☐ ☐
             1 2 3 4 5 6 7 8 9 10 .....

BREAKFAST	Calories	Carbs (g.)	Added Sugar (g.)	Fiber (g.)	Protein (g.)	Fat (g.)
Time *Total:*						

SNACK						
Time *Total:*						

LUNCH						
Time *Total:*						

DINNER						
Time *Total:*						

SNACK						
Time *Total:*						

VITAMINS/SUPPLEMENT/MEDS	Notes

DAYS______________ **DATE**________________________ **WEIGHT**________________

Sleep (Hrs) : ☐ ☐ ☐ ☐ ☐ ☐ ☐ ☐ ☐ ☐   Water (Cup) : ☐ ☐ ☐ ☐ ☐ ☐ ☐ ☐ ☐ ☐
         1 2 3 4 5 6 7 8 9 10 ....   1 2 3 4 5 6 7 8 9 10 ....

BREAKFAST	Calories	Carbs (g.)	Added Sugar (g.)	Fiber (g.)	Protein (g.)	Fat (g.)
Time	Total:					
SNACK						
Time	Total:					
LUNCH						
Time	Total:					
DINNER						
Time	Total:					
SNACK						
Time	Total:					

VITAMINS/SUPPLEMENT/MEDS	Notes

DAYS_________________**DATE**_________________________**WEIGHT**_________________

Sleep (Hrs) : ☐ ☐ ☐ ☐ ☐ ☐ ☐ ☐ ☐ ☐
         1 2 3 4 5 6 7 8 9 10 .....

Water (Cup) : ☐ ☐ ☐ ☐ ☐ ☐ ☐ ☐ ☐ ☐
           1 2 3 4 5 6 7 8 9 10 .....

BREAKFAST	Calories	Carbs (g.)	Added Sugar (g.)	Fiber (g.)	Protein (g.)	Fat (g.)
Time _____ Total:						
SNACK						
Time _____ Total:						
LUNCH						
Time _____ Total:						
DINNER						
Time _____ Total:						
SNACK						
Time _____ Total:						

VITAMINS/SUPPLEMENT/MEDS	Notes

DAYS______________________**DATE**________________________________ **WEIGHT**__________________

Sleep (Hrs) : ☐ ☐ ☐ ☐ ☐ ☐ ☐ ☐ ☐ ☐   Water (Cup) : ☐ ☐ ☐ ☐ ☐ ☐ ☐ ☐ ☐ ☐
1 2 3 4 5 6 7 8 9 10 .....   1 2 3 4 5 6 7 8 9 10 .....

BREAKFAST	Calories	Carbs (g.)	Added Sugar (g.)	Fiber (g.)	Protein (g.)	Fat (g.)
Time Total:						

SNACK						
Time Total:						

LUNCH						
Time Total:						

DINNER						
Time Total:						

SNACK						
Time Total:						

VITAMINS/SUPPLEMENT/MEDS	Notes

DAYS___________________**DATE**_______________________________**WEIGHT**_________________

Sleep (Hrs) : ☐ ☐ ☐ ☐ ☐ ☐ ☐ ☐ ☐ ☐
           1 2 3 4 5 6 7 8 9 10 .....

Water (Cup) : ☐ ☐ ☐ ☐ ☐ ☐ ☐ ☐ ☐ ☐
           1 2 3 4 5 6 7 8 9 10 .....

BREAKFAST	Calories	Carbs (g.)	Added Sugar (g.)	Fiber (g.)	Protein (g.)	Fat (g.)
Time *Total:*						
SNACK						
Time *Total:*						
LUNCH						
Time *Total:*						
DINNER						
Time *Total:*						
SNACK						
Time *Total:*						

VITAMINS/SUPPLEMENT/MEDS	Notes

DAYS__________________ **DATE**________________________________ **WEIGHT**________________

Sleep (Hrs) : ☐ ☐ ☐ ☐ ☐ ☐ ☐ ☐ ☐ ☐
1 2 3 4 5 6 7 8 9 10 .....

Water (Cup) : ☐ ☐ ☐ ☐ ☐ ☐ ☐ ☐ ☐ ☐
1 2 3 4 5 6 7 8 9 10 .....

BREAKFAST	Calories	Carbs (g.)	Added Sugar (g.)	Fiber (g.)	Protein (g.)	Fat (g.)
Time __________ Total:						
SNACK						
Time __________ Total:						
LUNCH						
Time __________ Total:						
DINNER						
Time __________ Total:						
SNACK						
Time __________ Total:						

VITAMINS/SUPPLEMENT/MEDS	Notes

DAYS_____________________**DATE**_______________________________**WEIGHT**_________________

Sleep (Hrs) : ☐ ☐ ☐ ☐ ☐ ☐ ☐ ☐ ☐ ☐   Water (Cup) : ☐ ☐ ☐ ☐ ☐ ☐ ☐ ☐ ☐ ☐
     1 2 3 4 5 6 7 8 9 10 .....   1 2 3 4 5 6 7 8 9 10 .....

BREAKFAST	Calories	Carbs (g.)	Added Sugar (g.)	Fiber (g.)	Protein (g.)	Fat (g.)
Time *Total:*						
SNACK						
Time *Total:*						
LUNCH						
Time *Total:*						
DINNER						
Time *Total:*						
SNACK						
Time *Total:*						

VITAMINS/SUPPLEMENT/MEDS	Notes

DAYS_______________ **DATE**_____________________________ **WEIGHT**_______________

Sleep (Hrs) : ☐ ☐ ☐ ☐ ☐ ☐ ☐ ☐ ☐ ☐ Water (Cup) : ☐ ☐ ☐ ☐ ☐ ☐ ☐ ☐ ☐ ☐
         1 2 3 4 5 6 7 8 9 10 .....   1 2 3 4 5 6 7 8 9 10 .....

BREAKFAST	Calories	Carbs (g.)	Added Sugar (g.)	Fiber (g.)	Protein (g.)	Fat (g.)
Time Total:						

SNACK						
Time Total:						

LUNCH						
Time Total:						

DINNER						
Time Total:						

SNACK						
Time Total:						

VITAMINS/SUPPLEMENT/MEDS	Notes

DAYS_________________**DATE**_______________________________**WEIGHT**________________

Sleep (Hrs) : ☐ ☐ ☐ ☐ ☐ ☐ ☐ ☐ ☐ ☐ .....
 1 2 3 4 5 6 7 8 9 10

Water (Cup) : ☐ ☐ ☐ ☐ ☐ ☐ ☐ ☐ ☐ ☐ .....
 1 2 3 4 5 6 7 8 9 10

BREAKFAST	Calories	Carbs (g.)	Added Sugar (g.)	Fiber (g.)	Protein (g.)	Fat (g.)
Time *Total:*						

SNACK						
Time *Total:*						

LUNCH						
Time *Total:*						

DINNER						
Time *Total:*						

SNACK						
Time *Total:*						

VITAMINS/SUPPLEMENT/MEDS	Notes

DAYS___________________ **DATE**___________________________________ **WEIGHT**_________________

Sleep (Hrs) : ☐ ☐ ☐ ☐ ☐ ☐ ☐ ☐ ☐ ☐
          1 2 3 4 5 6 7 8 9 10 .....

Water (Cup) : ☐ ☐ ☐ ☐ ☐ ☐ ☐ ☐ ☐ ☐
            1 2 3 4 5 6 7 8 9 10 .....

BREAKFAST	Calories	Carbs (g.)	Added Sugar (g.)	Fiber (g.)	Protein (g.)	Fat (g.)
Time *Total:*						
SNACK						
Time *Total:*						
LUNCH						
Time *Total:*						
DINNER						
Time *Total:*						
SNACK						
Time *Total:*						

VITAMINS/SUPPLEMENT/MEDS	Notes

DAYS__________________**DATE**___________________________________**WEIGHT**___________________

Sleep (Hrs) : ☐ ☐ ☐ ☐ ☐ ☐ ☐ ☐ ☐ ☐
1   2   3   4   5   6   7   8   9 10 .....

Water (Cup) : ☐ ☐ ☐ ☐ ☐ ☐ ☐ ☐ ☐ ☐
1   2   3   4   5   6   7   8   9 10 .....

BREAKFAST	Calories	Carbs (g.)	Added Sugar (g.)	Fiber (g.)	Protein (g.)	Fat (g.)
Time *Total:*						
SNACK						
Time *Total:*						
LUNCH						
Time *Total:*						
DINNER						
Time *Total:*						
SNACK						
Time *Total:*						

VITAMINS/SUPPLEMENT/MEDS	Notes

DAYS_________________ **DATE**_________________________________ **WEIGHT**__________________

Sleep (Hrs) : ☐ ☐ ☐ ☐ ☐ ☐ ☐ ☐ ☐ ☐
          1 2 3 4 5 6 7 8 9 10 .....   Water (Cup) : ☐ ☐ ☐ ☐ ☐ ☐ ☐ ☐ ☐ ☐
                                                      1 2 3 4 5 6 7 8 9 10 .....

BREAKFAST	Calories	Carbs (g.)	Added Sugar (g.)	Fiber (g.)	Protein (g.)	Fat (g.)
Time *Total:*						
SNACK						
Time *Total:*						
LUNCH						
Time *Total:*						
DINNER						
Time *Total:*						
SNACK						
Time *Total:*						

VITAMINS/SUPPLEMENT/MEDS	**Notes**

DAYS______________________**DATE**________________________________**WEIGHT**__________________

Sleep (Hrs) : ☐ ☐ ☐ ☐ ☐ ☐ ☐ ☐ ☐ ☐   Water (Cup) : ☐ ☐ ☐ ☐ ☐ ☐ ☐ ☐ ☐ ☐
1 2 3 4 5 6 7 8 9 10 .....   1 2 3 4 5 6 7 8 9 10 .....

BREAKFAST	Calories	Carbs (g.)	Added Sugar (g.)	Fiber (g.)	Protein (g.)	Fat (g.)
Time *Total:*						
SNACK						
Time *Total:*						
LUNCH						
Time *Total:*						
DINNER						
Time *Total:*						
SNACK						
Time *Total:*						

VITAMINS/SUPPLEMENT/MEDS	Notes

DAYS_______________**DATE**_______________________________**WEIGHT**_______________

Sleep (Hrs) : ☐ ☐ ☐ ☐ ☐ ☐ ☐ ☐ ☐ ☐   Water (Cup) : ☐ ☐ ☐ ☐ ☐ ☐ ☐ ☐ ☐ ☐
1 2 3 4 5 6 7 8 9 10 .....   1 2 3 4 5 6 7 8 9 10 .....

BREAKFAST	Calories	Carbs (g.)	Added Sugar (g.)	Fiber (g.)	Protein (g.)	Fat (g.)
Time *Total:*						

SNACK						
Time *Total:*						

LUNCH						
Time *Total:*						

DINNER						
Time *Total:*						

SNACK						
Time *Total:*						

VITAMINS/SUPPLEMENT/MEDS	Notes

DAYS____________________**DATE**____________________________________**WEIGHT**__________________

Sleep (Hrs) : ☐ ☐ ☐ ☐ ☐ ☐ ☐ ☐ ☐ ☐
          1 2 3 4 5 6 7 8 9 10 .....

Water (Cup) : ☐ ☐ ☐ ☐ ☐ ☐ ☐ ☐ ☐ ☐
           1 2 3 4 5 6 7 8 9 10 .....

BREAKFAST	Calories	Carbs (g.)	Added Sugar (g.)	Fiber (g.)	Protein (g.)	Fat (g.)
Time Total:						
SNACK						
Time Total:						
LUNCH						
Time Total:						
DINNER						
Time Total:						
SNACK						
Time Total:						

VITAMINS/SUPPLEMENT/MEDS	Notes

DAYS___________________ **DATE**_______________________________ **WEIGHT**___________________

Sleep (Hrs) : ☐ ☐ ☐ ☐ ☐ ☐ ☐ ☐ ☐ ☐   Water (Cup) : ☐ ☐ ☐ ☐ ☐ ☐ ☐ ☐ ☐ ☐
        1   2   3   4   5   6   7   8   9   10 ……   1   2   3   4   5   6   7   8   9   10 ……

BREAKFAST	Calories	Carbs (g.)	Added Sugar (g.)	Fiber (g.)	Protein (g.)	Fat (g.)
Time　　　　　　　*Total:*						
SNACK						
Time　　　　　　　*Total:*						
LUNCH						
Time　　　　　　　*Total:*						
DINNER						
Time　　　　　　　*Total:*						
SNACK						
Time　　　　　　　*Total:*						

VITAMINS/SUPPLEMENT/MEDS	Notes

DAYS_____________________**DATE**_____________________________**WEIGHT**_________________

Sleep (Hrs) : ☐ ☐ ☐ ☐ ☐ ☐ ☐ ☐ ☐ ☐
           1   2   3   4   5   6   7   8   9   10 .....

Water (Cup) : ☐ ☐ ☐ ☐ ☐ ☐ ☐ ☐ ☐ ☐
            1   2   3   4   5   6   7   8   9   10 .....

BREAKFAST	Calories	Carbs (g.)	Added Sugar (g.)	Fiber (g.)	Protein (g.)	Fat (g.)
Time *Total:*						

SNACK						
Time *Total:*						

LUNCH						
Time *Total:*						

DINNER						
Time *Total:*						

SNACK						
Time *Total:*						

VITAMINS/SUPPLEMENT/MEDS	Notes

DAYS_______________ **DATE**_______________________ **WEIGHT**_______________

Sleep (Hrs) : ☐ ☐ ☐ ☐ ☐ ☐ ☐ ☐ ☐ ☐
           1 2 3 4 5 6 7 8 9 10 .....

Water (Cup) : ☐ ☐ ☐ ☐ ☐ ☐ ☐ ☐ ☐ ☐
            1 2 3 4 5 6 7 8 9 10 .....

BREAKFAST	Calories	Carbs (g.)	Added Sugar (g.)	Fiber (g.)	Protein (g.)	Fat (g.)
Time	Total:					

SNACK						
Time	Total:					

LUNCH						
Time	Total:					

DINNER						
Time	Total:					

SNACK						
Time	Total:					

VITAMINS/SUPPLEMENT/MEDS	Notes

DAYS___________________**DATE**___________________________**WEIGHT**_________________

Sleep (Hrs) : ☐ ☐ ☐ ☐ ☐ ☐ ☐ ☐ ☐ ☐   Water (Cup) : ☐ ☐ ☐ ☐ ☐ ☐ ☐ ☐ ☐ ☐
       1 2 3 4 5 6 7 8 9 10 .....   1 2 3 4 5 6 7 8 9 10 .....

BREAKFAST	Calories	Carbs (g.)	Added Sugar (g.)	Fiber (g.)	Protein (g.)	Fat (g.)
Time *Total:*						
SNACK						
Time *Total:*						
LUNCH						
Time *Total:*						
DINNER						
Time *Total:*						
SNACK						
Time *Total:*						

VITAMINS/SUPPLEMENT/MEDS	Notes

DAYS___________________ **DATE**___________________________________ **WEIGHT**_______________

Sleep (Hrs) : ☐ ☐ ☐ ☐ ☐ ☐ ☐ ☐ ☐ ☐
 1 2 3 4 5 6 7 8 9 10 .....

Water (Cup) : ☐ ☐ ☐ ☐ ☐ ☐ ☐ ☐ ☐ ☐
 1 2 3 4 5 6 7 8 9 10 .....

BREAKFAST	Calories	Carbs (g.)	Added Sugar (g.)	Fiber (g.)	Protein (g.)	Fat (g.)
Time　　　　　　　　*Total:*						
SNACK						
Time　　　　　　　　*Total:*						
LUNCH						
Time　　　　　　　　*Total:*						
DINNER						
Time　　　　　　　　*Total:*						
SNACK						
Time　　　　　　　　*Total:*						

VITAMINS/SUPPLEMENT/MEDS	Notes

DAYS______________ **DATE**______________________ **WEIGHT**______________

Sleep (Hrs) : ☐ ☐ ☐ ☐ ☐ ☐ ☐ ☐ ☐ ☐
          1   2   3   4   5   6   7   8   9   10 .....

Water (Cup) : ☐ ☐ ☐ ☐ ☐ ☐ ☐ ☐ ☐ ☐
          1   2   3   4   5   6   7   8   9   10 .....

BREAKFAST	Calories	Carbs (g.)	Added Sugar (g.)	Fiber (g.)	Protein (g.)	Fat (g.)
Time _______ Total:						

SNACK						
Time _______ Total:						

LUNCH						
Time _______ Total:						

DINNER						
Time _______ Total:						

SNACK						
Time _______ Total:						

VITAMINS/SUPPLEMENT/MEDS	Notes

DAYS__________________ **DATE**____________________________ **WEIGHT**________________

Sleep (Hrs) : ☐ ☐ ☐ ☐ ☐ ☐ ☐ ☐ ☐ ☐   Water (Cup) : ☐ ☐ ☐ ☐ ☐ ☐ ☐ ☐ ☐ ☐
          1 2 3 4 5 6 7 8 9 10 .....   1 2 3 4 5 6 7 8 9 10 .....

BREAKFAST	Calories	Carbs (g.)	Added Sugar (g.)	Fiber (g.)	Protein (g.)	Fat (g.)
Time *Total:*						
SNACK						
Time *Total:*						
LUNCH						
Time *Total:*						
DINNER						
Time *Total:*						
SNACK						
Time *Total:*						

VITAMINS/SUPPLEMENT/MEDS	Notes

DAYS_____________________ **DATE**_________________________________ **WEIGHT**_______________

Sleep (Hrs) : ☐ ☐ ☐ ☐ ☐ ☐ ☐ ☐ ☐ ☐ .....   Water (Cup) : ☐ ☐ ☐ ☐ ☐ ☐ ☐ ☐ ☐ ☐ .....
             1 2 3 4 5 6 7 8 9 10   1 2 3 4 5 6 7 8 9 10

BREAKFAST	Calories	Carbs (g.)	Added Sugar (g.)	Fiber (g.)	Protein (g.)	Fat (g.)
Time *Total:*						
SNACK						
Time *Total:*						
LUNCH						
Time *Total:*						
DINNER						
Time *Total:*						
SNACK						
Time *Total:*						

VITAMINS/SUPPLEMENT/MEDS	Notes

DAYS_____________________**DATE**_____________________________**WEIGHT**___________________

Sleep (Hrs) : ☐ ☐ ☐ ☐ ☐ ☐ ☐ ☐ ☐ ☐
          1 2 3 4 5 6 7 8 9 10 ....

Water (Cup) : ☐ ☐ ☐ ☐ ☐ ☐ ☐ ☐ ☐ ☐
          1 2 3 4 5 6 7 8 9 10 ....

BREAKFAST	Calories	Carbs (g.)	Added Sugar (g.)	Fiber (g.)	Protein (g.)	Fat (g.)
Time _______ Total:						

SNACK						
Time _______ Total:						

LUNCH						
Time _______ Total:						

DINNER						
Time _______ Total:						

SNACK						
Time _______ Total:						

VITAMINS/SUPPLEMENT/MEDS	Notes

DAYS___________________**DATE**_______________________________**WEIGHT**________________

Sleep (Hrs) : ☐ ☐ ☐ ☐ ☐ ☐ ☐ ☐ ☐ ☐   Water (Cup) : ☐ ☐ ☐ ☐ ☐ ☐ ☐ ☐ ☐ ☐
1 2 3 4 5 6 7 8 9 10 .....   1 2 3 4 5 6 7 8 9 10 .....

BREAKFAST	Calories	Carbs (g.)	Added Sugar (g.)	Fiber (g.)	Protein (g.)	Fat (g.)
Time *Total:*						
SNACK						
Time *Total:*						
LUNCH						
Time *Total:*						
DINNER						
Time *Total:*						
SNACK						
Time *Total:*						

VITAMINS/SUPPLEMENT/MEDS	Notes

DAYS______________ **DATE**________________________ **WEIGHT**______________

Sleep (Hrs) : ☐ ☐ ☐ ☐ ☐ ☐ ☐ ☐ ☐ ☐
             1 2 3 4 5 6 7 8 9 10 .....

Water (Cup) : ☐ ☐ ☐ ☐ ☐ ☐ ☐ ☐ ☐ ☐
             1 2 3 4 5 6 7 8 9 10 .....

BREAKFAST	Calories	Carbs (g.)	Added Sugar (g.)	Fiber (g.)	Protein (g.)	Fat (g.)
Time *Total:*						

SNACK						
Time *Total:*						

LUNCH						
Time *Total:*						

DINNER						
Time *Total:*						

SNACK						
Time *Total:*						

VITAMINS/SUPPLEMENT/MEDS	Notes

DAYS_______________**DATE**_______________________________**WEIGHT**_______________

Sleep (Hrs) : ☐ ☐ ☐ ☐ ☐ ☐ ☐ ☐ ☐ ☐
          1 2 3 4 5 6 7 8 9 10 .....
Water (Cup) : ☐ ☐ ☐ ☐ ☐ ☐ ☐ ☐ ☐ ☐
          1 2 3 4 5 6 7 8 9 10 .....

BREAKFAST	Calories	Carbs (g.)	Added Sugar (g.)	Fiber (g.)	Protein (g.)	Fat (g.)
Time *Total:*						
SNACK						
Time *Total:*						
LUNCH						
Time *Total:*						
DINNER						
Time *Total:*						
SNACK						
Time *Total:*						

VITAMINS/SUPPLEMENT/MEDS	Notes

DAYS_______________ **DATE**_________________________________ **WEIGHT**_________________

Sleep (Hrs) : ☐ ☐ ☐ ☐ ☐ ☐ ☐ ☐ ☐ ☐
          1 2 3 4 5 6 7 8 9 10 .....

Water (Cup) : ☐ ☐ ☐ ☐ ☐ ☐ ☐ ☐ ☐ ☐
          1 2 3 4 5 6 7 8 9 10 .....

BREAKFAST	Calories	Carbs (g.)	Added Sugar (g.)	Fiber (g.)	Protein (g.)	Fat (g.)
Time *Total:*						
SNACK						
Time *Total:*						
LUNCH						
Time *Total:*						
DINNER						
Time *Total:*						
SNACK						
Time *Total:*						

VITAMINS/SUPPLEMENT/MEDS	Notes

DAYS__________________ **DATE**_________________________________ **WEIGHT**___________________

Sleep (Hrs) : ☐ ☐ ☐ ☐ ☐ ☐ ☐ ☐ ☐ ☐
　　　　　　　1　2　3　4　5　6　7　8　9　10 .....

Water (Cup) : ☐ ☐ ☐ ☐ ☐ ☐ ☐ ☐ ☐ ☐
　　　　　　　1　2　3　4　5　6　7　8　9　10 .....

BREAKFAST	Calories	Carbs (g.)	Added Sugar (g.)	Fiber (g.)	Protein (g.)	Fat (g.)
Time　　　　　　　*Total:*						

SNACK						
Time　　　　　　　*Total:*						

LUNCH						
Time　　　　　　　*Total:*						

DINNER						
Time　　　　　　　*Total:*						

SNACK						
Time　　　　　　　*Total:*						

VITAMINS/SUPPLEMENT/MEDS	Notes

DAYS_______________________ **DATE**____ **WEIGHT**__________________________

Sleep (Hrs) : ☐ ☐ ☐ ☐ ☐ ☐ ☐ ☐ ☐ ☐
            1 2 3 4 5 6 7 8 9 10 .....

Water (Cup) : ☐ ☐ ☐ ☐ ☐ ☐ ☐ ☐ ☐ ☐
              1 2 3 4 5 6 7 8 9 10 .....

BREAKFAST	Calories	Carbs (g.)	Added Sugar (g.)	Fiber (g.)	Protein (g.)	Fat (g.)
Time *Total:*						
SNACK						
Time *Total:*						
LUNCH						
Time *Total:*						
DINNER						
Time *Total:*						
SNACK						
Time *Total:*						

VITAMINS/SUPPLEMENT/MEDS	Notes

DAYS______________________**DATE**______________________________ **WEIGHT**______________________

Sleep (Hrs) : ☐ ☐ ☐ ☐ ☐ ☐ ☐ ☐ ☐ ☐
           1 2 3 4 5 6 7 8 9 10 .....

Water (Cup) : ☐ ☐ ☐ ☐ ☐ ☐ ☐ ☐ ☐ ☐
            1 2 3 4 5 6 7 8 9 10 .....

BREAKFAST	Calories	Carbs (g.)	Added Sugar (g.)	Fiber (g.)	Protein (g.)	Fat (g.)
Time *Total:*						
SNACK						
Time *Total:*						
LUNCH						
Time *Total:*						
DINNER						
Time *Total:*						
SNACK						
Time *Total:*						

VITAMINS/SUPPLEMENT/MEDS	**Notes**

DAYS_________________ **DATE**_____________________________ **WEIGHT**_________________

Sleep (Hrs) : ☐ ☐ ☐ ☐ ☐ ☐ ☐ ☐ ☐ ☐
          1 2 3 4 5 6 7 8 9 10 .....

Water (Cup) : ☐ ☐ ☐ ☐ ☐ ☐ ☐ ☐ ☐ ☐
          1 2 3 4 5 6 7 8 9 10 .....

BREAKFAST	Calories	Carbs (g.)	Added Sugar (g.)	Fiber (g.)	Protein (g.)	Fat (g.)
Time *Total:*						
SNACK						
Time *Total:*						
LUNCH						
Time *Total:*						
DINNER						
Time *Total:*						
SNACK						
Time *Total:*						

VITAMINS/SUPPLEMENT/MEDS	Notes

DAYS__________________**DATE**__________________________________**WEIGHT**__________________

Sleep (Hrs) : ☐ ☐ ☐ ☐ ☐ ☐ ☐ ☐ ☐ ☐
           1 2 3 4 5 6 7 8 9 10 .....

Water (Cup) : ☐ ☐ ☐ ☐ ☐ ☐ ☐ ☐ ☐ ☐
           1 2 3 4 5 6 7 8 9 10 .....

BREAKFAST	Calories	Carbs (g.)	Added Sugar (g.)	Fiber (g.)	Protein (g.)	Fat (g.)
Time *Total:*						
SNACK						
Time *Total:*						
LUNCH						
Time *Total:*						
DINNER						
Time *Total:*						
SNACK						
Time *Total:*						

VITAMINS/SUPPLEMENT/MEDS	Notes

DAYS_____________________ **DATE**_____________________________________ **WEIGHT**_____________________

Sleep (Hrs) : ☐ ☐ ☐ ☐ ☐ ☐ ☐ ☐ ☐ ☐ ......
          1   2   3   4   5   6   7   8   9   10

Water (Cup) : ☐ ☐ ☐ ☐ ☐ ☐ ☐ ☐ ☐ ☐ ......
          1   2   3   4   5   6   7   8   9   10

BREAKFAST	Calories	Carbs (g.)	Added Sugar (g.)	Fiber (g.)	Protein (g.)	Fat (g.)
Time Total:						
SNACK						
Time Total:						
LUNCH						
Time Total:						
DINNER						
Time Total:						
SNACK						
Time Total:						

VITAMINS/SUPPLEMENT/MEDS	**Notes**

DAYS_____________________**DATE**_________________________________**WEIGHT**________________________

Sleep (Hrs) : ☐ ☐ ☐ ☐ ☐ ☐ ☐ ☐ ☐ ☐   Water (Cup) : ☐ ☐ ☐ ☐ ☐ ☐ ☐ ☐ ☐ ☐
 1 2 3 4 5 6 7 8 9 10 .....   1 2 3 4 5 6 7 8 9 10 .....

BREAKFAST	Calories	Carbs (g.)	Added Sugar (g.)	Fiber (g.)	Protein (g.)	Fat (g.)
Time *Total:*						

SNACK						
Time *Total:*						

LUNCH						
Time *Total:*						

DINNER						
Time *Total:*						

SNACK						
Time *Total:*						

VITAMINS/SUPPLEMENT/MEDS	Notes

DAYS_________________ **DATE**_________________________________ **WEIGHT**________________

Sleep (Hrs) : ☐ ☐ ☐ ☐ ☐ ☐ ☐ ☐ ☐ ☐
        1 2 3 4 5 6 7 8 9 10 .....

Water (Cup) : ☐ ☐ ☐ ☐ ☐ ☐ ☐ ☐ ☐ ☐
        1 2 3 4 5 6 7 8 9 10 .....

BREAKFAST	Calories	Carbs (g.)	Added Sugar (g.)	Fiber (g.)	Protein (g.)	Fat (g.)
Time *Total:*						
SNACK						
Time *Total:*						
LUNCH						
Time *Total:*						
DINNER						
Time *Total:*						
SNACK						
Time *Total:*						

VITAMINS/SUPPLEMENT/MEDS	Notes

DAYS_________________ **DATE**_______________________________ **WEIGHT**___________________

Sleep (Hrs) : ☐ ☐ ☐ ☐ ☐ ☐ ☐ ☐ ☐ ☐   Water (Cup) : ☐ ☐ ☐ ☐ ☐ ☐ ☐ ☐ ☐ ☐
        1 2 3 4 5 6 7 8 9 10 ....   1 2 3 4 5 6 7 8 9 10 ....

BREAKFAST	Calories	Carbs (g.)	Added Sugar (g.)	Fiber (g.)	Protein (g.)	Fat (g.)
Time *Total:*						
SNACK						
Time *Total:*						
LUNCH						
Time *Total:*						
DINNER						
Time *Total:*						
SNACK						
Time *Total:*						

VITAMINS/SUPPLEMENT/MEDS	Notes

DAYS______________**DATE**________________________________**WEIGHT**________________

Sleep (Hrs) : ☐ ☐ ☐ ☐ ☐ ☐ ☐ ☐ ☐ ☐ Water (Cup) : ☐ ☐ ☐ ☐ ☐ ☐ ☐ ☐ ☐ ☐
        1 2 3 4 5 6 7 8 9 10 .....   1 2 3 4 5 6 7 8 9 10 .....

BREAKFAST	Calories	Carbs (g.)	Added Sugar (g.)	Fiber (g.)	Protein (g.)	Fat (g.)
Time *Total:*						

SNACK						
Time *Total:*						

LUNCH						
Time *Total:*						

DINNER						
Time *Total:*						

SNACK						
Time *Total:*						

VITAMINS/SUPPLEMENT/MEDS	Notes

DAYS_____________________**DATE**_________________________________**WEIGHT**_____________________

Sleep (Hrs) : ☐ ☐ ☐ ☐ ☐ ☐ ☐ ☐ ☐ ☐
            1 2 3 4 5 6 7 8 9 10 .....

Water (Cup) : ☐ ☐ ☐ ☐ ☐ ☐ ☐ ☐ ☐ ☐
            1 2 3 4 5 6 7 8 9 10 .....

BREAKFAST	Calories	Carbs (g.)	Added Sugar (g.)	Fiber (g.)	Protein (g.)	Fat (g.)
Time Total:						
SNACK						
Time Total:						
LUNCH						
Time Total:						
DINNER						
Time Total:						
SNACK						
Time Total:						

VITAMINS/SUPPLEMENT/MEDS	Notes

DAYS_________________ **DATE**____________________________ **WEIGHT**________________

Sleep (Hrs) : ☐ ☐ ☐ ☐ ☐ ☐ ☐ ☐ ☐ ☐
        1   2   3   4   5   6   7   8   9   10 .....

Water (Cup) : ☐ ☐ ☐ ☐ ☐ ☐ ☐ ☐ ☐ ☐
        1   2   3   4   5   6   7   8   9   10 .....

BREAKFAST	Calories	Carbs (g.)	Added Sugar (g.)	Fiber (g.)	Protein (g.)	Fat (g.)
Time *Total:*						

SNACK						
Time *Total:*						

LUNCH						
Time *Total:*						

DINNER						
Time *Total:*						

SNACK						
Time *Total:*						

VITAMINS/SUPPLEMENT/MEDS	Notes

DAYS___________________**DATE**_______________________________**WEIGHT**___________________

Sleep (Hrs) : ☐ ☐ ☐ ☐ ☐ ☐ ☐ ☐ ☐ ☐
            1 2 3 4 5 6 7 8 9 10 .....

Water (Cup) : ☐ ☐ ☐ ☐ ☐ ☐ ☐ ☐ ☐ ☐
            1 2 3 4 5 6 7 8 9 10 .....

BREAKFAST	Calories	Carbs (g.)	Added Sugar (g.)	Fiber (g.)	Protein (g.)	Fat (g.)
Time *Total:*						
SNACK						
Time *Total:*						
LUNCH						
Time *Total:*						
DINNER						
Time *Total:*						
SNACK						
Time *Total:*						

VITAMINS/SUPPLEMENT/MEDS	Notes

DAYS_________________ **DATE**_________________________________ **WEIGHT**___________________

Sleep (Hrs) : ☐ ☐ ☐ ☐ ☐ ☐ ☐ ☐ ☐ ☐ ....
　　　　　　　1　2　3　4　5　6　7　8　9　10

Water (Cup) : ☐ ☐ ☐ ☐ ☐ ☐ ☐ ☐ ☐ ☐ ....
　　　　　　　　1　2　3　4　5　6　7　8　9　10

BREAKFAST	Calories	Carbs (g.)	Added Sugar (g.)	Fiber (g.)	Protein (g.)	Fat (g.)
Time Total:						

SNACK						
Time Total:						

LUNCH						
Time Total:						

DINNER						
Time Total:						

SNACK						
Time Total:						

VITAMINS/SUPPLEMENT/MEDS	Notes

DAYS___________________**DATE**___________________________**WEIGHT**_________________

Sleep (Hrs) : ☐ ☐ ☐ ☐ ☐ ☐ ☐ ☐ ☐ ☐   Water (Cup) : ☐ ☐ ☐ ☐ ☐ ☐ ☐ ☐ ☐ ☐
       1   2   3   4   5   6   7   8   9   10   1   2   3   4   5   6   7   8   9   10 .....

BREAKFAST	Calories	Carbs (g.)	Added Sugar (g.)	Fiber (g.)	Protein (g.)	Fat (g.)
Time Total:						
SNACK						
Time Total:						
LUNCH						
Time Total:						
DINNER						
Time Total:						
SNACK						
Time Total:						

VITAMINS/SUPPLEMENT/MEDS	Notes

DAYS_________________ **DATE**_________________________________ **WEIGHT**_________________

Sleep (Hrs) : ☐ ☐ ☐ ☐ ☐ ☐ ☐ ☐ ☐ ☐ Water (Cup) : ☐ ☐ ☐ ☐ ☐ ☐ ☐ ☐ ☐ ☐
1 2 3 4 5 6 7 8 9 10 .....   1 2 3 4 5 6 7 8 9 10 .....

BREAKFAST	Calories	Carbs (g.)	Added Sugar (g.)	Fiber (g.)	Protein (g.)	Fat (g.)
Time	Total:					
SNACK						
Time	Total:					
LUNCH						
Time	Total:					
DINNER						
Time	Total:					
SNACK						
Time	Total:					

VITAMINS/SUPPLEMENT/MEDS	Notes

DAYS___________________**DATE**___________________________**WEIGHT**___________________

Sleep (Hrs) : ☐ ☐ ☐ ☐ ☐ ☐ ☐ ☐ ☐ ☐   Water (Cup) : ☐ ☐ ☐ ☐ ☐ ☐ ☐ ☐ ☐ ☐
       1 2 3 4 5 6 7 8 9 10 .....   1 2 3 4 5 6 7 8 9 10 .....

BREAKFAST	Calories	Carbs (g.)	Added Sugar (g.)	Fiber (g.)	Protein (g.)	Fat (g.)
Time *Total:*						
SNACK						
Time *Total:*						
LUNCH						
Time *Total:*						
DINNER						
Time *Total:*						
SNACK						
Time *Total:*						

VITAMINS/SUPPLEMENT/MEDS	Notes

DAYS______________________**DATE**______________________________**WEIGHT**______________________

Sleep (Hrs) : ☐ ☐ ☐ ☐ ☐ ☐ ☐ ☐ ☐ ☐
1　2　3　4　5　6　7　8　9　10 .....

Water (Cup) : ☐ ☐ ☐ ☐ ☐ ☐ ☐ ☐ ☐ ☐
1　2　3　4　5　6　7　8　9　10 .....

BREAKFAST	Calories	Carbs (g.)	Added Sugar (g.)	Fiber (g.)	Protein (g.)	Fat (g.)
Time *Total:*						
SNACK						
Time *Total:*						
LUNCH						
Time *Total:*						
DINNER						
Time *Total:*						
SNACK						
Time *Total:*						

VITAMINS/SUPPLEMENT/MEDS	Notes

Sleep (Hrs) : ☐ ☐ ☐ ☐ ☐ ☐ ☐ ☐ ☐ ☐
            1 2 3 4 5 6 7 8 9 10 .....

Water (Cup) : ☐ ☐ ☐ ☐ ☐ ☐ ☐ ☐ ☐ ☐
            1 2 3 4 5 6 7 8 9 10 .....

BREAKFAST	Calories	Carbs (g.)	Added Sugar (g.)	Fiber (g.)	Protein (g.)	Fat (g.)
Time *Total:*						
SNACK						
Time *Total:*						
LUNCH						
Time *Total:*						
DINNER						
Time *Total:*						
SNACK						
Time *Total:*						

VITAMINS/SUPPLEMENT/MEDS	Notes

DAYS_________________ **DATE**_________________________________ **WEIGHT**___________________

Sleep (Hrs) : ☐ ☐ ☐ ☐ ☐ ☐ ☐ ☐ ☐ ☐
         1 2 3 4 5 6 7 8 9 10 .....

Water (Cup) : ☐ ☐ ☐ ☐ ☐ ☐ ☐ ☐ ☐ ☐
         1 2 3 4 5 6 7 8 9 10 .....

BREAKFAST	Calories	Carbs (g.)	Added Sugar (g.)	Fiber (g.)	Protein (g.)	Fat (g.)
Time *Total:*						
SNACK						
Time *Total:*						
LUNCH						
Time *Total:*						
DINNER						
Time *Total:*						
SNACK						
Time *Total:*						

VITAMINS/SUPPLEMENT/MEDS	Notes

Notes

Notes

Notes

Notes